Podiatry
For
The
Reflexologist

Podiatric Pathology That Every Reflexologist Should Know

By Dr. Michelle Soble, D.P.M.
medicalreflexology@hotmail.com
www.drshelly.net

Call 1-866-DRSOBLE (377-6253) or visit
www.drshelly.net to inquire about book orders,
consultations and seminars. Or write to:

Dr. Michelle Soble, D.P.M.
P.O. Box 251413
West Bloomfield, MI 48325

Copyright 2002
Dr. Michelle Soble, D.P.M., PC
All rights reserved. No part of this book may be reproduced without
written consent from the publisher.

Library of Congress Cataloguing in Publication Data
Michelle Soble, D.P.M., PC

Manufactured in the United States of America
ISBN 0-9721877-0-7

Acknowledgements

I am grateful to my editor, Christina Job. Her knowledge and expertise is greatly appreciated.

Thank you to my husband David and my children Noah and Zoe for their patience and support.

Thank you to my parents Irv and Doreen Lichtman and my inlaws Ken and Doree Soble for their encouragement and love.

Thank you to my patients for giving me the gift to treat all of you and for helping me discover new challenges.

A special thank you to Bill and Kay Jean Furlong, founders of the Reflexology Association of Illinois, for inspiring me to write this book.

I dedicate this book to my father, Irving Lichtman, who has perfect feet.

ABOUT THE AUTHOR

Michelle Soble, D.P.M. is a podiatrist and a reflexologist. She practices Medical Reflexologysm in West Bloomfield, Michigan.

As a podiatrist, Dr. Soble treated homebound, closed head injury and special needs patients. She focused her studies on diabetic and vascular diseases. Dr. Soble was the 1992 recipient of the Ralph White Award for providing exceptional diabetic foot care.

As a podiatrist and reflexologist, Dr. Soble, promotes reflexology as a complimentary medical modality through television news media, seminars and publications.

Dr. Soble believes that western medicine is just beginning to learn about the substantial health benefits from reflexology.

Contents

INTRODUCTION

As a practicing podiatrist and reflexologist, my medical knowledge has been the key to achieving successful results for my reflexology patients. It is important all reflexologists learn about medical conditions affecting the feet.

My purpose in writing this book is to teach reflexologists to understand and recognize common podiatric problems they will most likely see in their practice. This book includes many podiatric pathologies that develop from systemic diseases. For most conditions, I include a description of the problem, followed by the cause, signs and symptoms, treatment, prevention and reflexology suggestions. I also share my own clinical experience and results using reflexology.

The treatments described in this book are conventional medical treatments that medical doctors may use to treat the stated condition. A reflexologist should use this book for recognizing and understanding conditions that affect the feet, <u>not for diagnostic purposes.</u>

After reading this book, you will gain the ability to identify common foot pathologies podiatrists/reflexologists see everyday. It is my hope that with this knowledge both your reflexology practice and the profession as a whole will be enhanced.

CHAPTER 1

ANATOMY

ANATOMY

Bones (picture1)

Each foot and ankle has 26 bones, together both feet and ankles contain a quarter of all the bones in the entire body.

Each foot is divided into three main parts: forefoot, midfoot and hindfoot.

Forefoot

The forefoot contains 14 phalanx bones that comprise the digits (toes). Connecting the toes to the midfoot are five metatarsal bones. Located on the plantar aspect of the hallux (big toe) are two sesamoid bones that allow the hallux to dorsiflex and plantarflex. The forefoot bears half the body's weight and absorbs pressure on the ball of the foot.

Midfoot

The midfoot consists of five tarsal bones and forms the arch of the foot. The five bones are the three cuniforms, the navicular and the cuboid bone.

The midfoot absorbs shock and is attached to the forefoot and hindfoot by muscles and fascia.

Hindfoot

There are two bones that form the hindfoot. They are the

talus and calcaneus. The talus connects the foot to the leg and allows the foot to plantarflex and dorsiflex.

The calcaneus is the heel bone; it is the largest bone in the foot. It forms a joint with the talus bone and allows the ankle to rotate. The plantar aspect of the heel is cushioned with plantar fat, which aids in shock absorption during gait (walking).

<u>Muscles, Tendons, Ligaments, Nerves and Blood Vessels</u>

Muscles, tendons and ligaments support the many bones in the feet and help shape the arch. In each foot there are 33 joints, 107 ligaments, 20 muscles, 125,000 sweat glands and over 7,000 nerve endings.

Main muscles of the foot:

Anterior tibial: allows the foot to dorsiflex and plantarflex (move up and down)

Posterior tibial: supports the arch

Peroneal: allows lateral ankle movement

Extensors: dorsiflex digits (point toes upward)

Flexors: plantarflex digits (point toes downward)

The achilles tendon is the largest and strongest tendon that extends from the calf to the heel.

Ligaments hold tendons in place and are a joint stabilizer.

The plantar fascia is a band of tissue that originates on the plantar aspect of the calcaneous bone and inserts at the ball of the foot. The plantar fascia helps to form the arch of the foot.

The sciatic nerve branches into the tibial and common peroneal nerves which are the main nerve supply to the feet. The tibial nerve branches into the medial and lateral plantar nerves. The common peroneal nerve branches into the superficial and deep peroneal nerves.

The arterial supply to the feet is from the femoral artery. The femoral artery becomes the popliteal artery. The popliteal artery branches into the anterior tibial artery and the posterior tibial artery. The anterior tibial artery becomes the dorsalis pedis artery and the lateral plantar artery. The posterior tibial artery becomes the medial plantar artery.

CHAPTER 2

NAIL PATHOLOGY

NAILS (picture 2)

The appearance of the nail plate can be a diagnostic tool for many medical conditions. Nail abnormalities are based on shape, color, texture and thickness. Nails, made of a protein called keratin, grow an average of 0.1 millimeters each day. However, growth rate is affected by disease, hormones and aging. Nail disorders are common and account for 10 percent of all skin conditions.

A nail consists of many parts:

Nailplate: the part of the nail that you see.

Nailbed: the skin under the nail plate.

Matrix: the area under the cuticle, where the nail grows

Lunula: the white half-moon shape at the base of the nail.

Cuticle: the tissue at the base of the nail that helps to protect against infection. To avoid infection never remove the cuticle.

Nailfolds: the folds of the skin that support the nail.

NAIL PATHOLOGY

Onychomycosis (picture 3)

Onychomycosis is a fungal infection of the nails. Fungus digests keratin. In response the body produces more keratin. An excess of keratin causes the nailplate to separate from the nailbed and become thick.

- Causes

Onychomycosis may be due to hereditary factors or trauma. It may also be a symptom of a disease process. Side effects from the following medications may cause fungus nails:

Bleomycin, Doxorubicin, 5-Fluorouracil, Retinoids, Captopril, Chlorpromazine, Chloramphenicol, Tetracyclines, Quinine and diuretics

- Signs and symptoms

The nailplate will become discolored, changing from a normal coloration to a yellow or brown color. The nailplate may become dystrophic, thick and crumbly, and become onycholytic (loosen from the nailbed). The nail may become painful due to pressure from the shoe and may also have an odor.

- Treatment

A podiatrist may suggest a topical anti-fungal cream, lotion or tincture to apply to the nailplate twice a day. Oral anti-fungal medication may be prescribed, however usage needs to be monitored due to serious side effects. Surgical removal of the toenail, using a chemical to destroy the cells that make the nail grow, is an option. Proper nail care, including nail debridement (trimming), is recommended.

- Prevention

Fungus thrives in dark, warm, moist environments, therefore preventing these factors are important. White 100 percent cotton socks and changing socks twice daily will decrease perspiration. After bathing or swimming, always dry feet completely to prevent a moist environment. Wear sandals in public bathing areas and increase the immune system through vitamins and a balanced diet.

Other nail abnormalities that may mimic fungus infections are:

psoriasis, lichen planus, contact dermatitis, yellow nail syndrome, candida (yeast infections).

Onychomycosis rarely occurs in children unless they are immunocompromised or have some form of cancer.

Nail Discolorations

Many systemic problems cause nail discolorations. Following is a list of different nail color changes and the possible causative factors:

Green Nails (Green Nail Syndrome)

- Causes

Pseudomonas, Aspergillus and Blastomyces infections

White Nails

- Causes

Autoimmune disorders, cardiac, gastrointestinal, renal and liver diseases, metabolic problems, neoplasia, psoriasis, stress, and trauma.

Black or Brown Nails

- Causes

Melanoma, nevi and trauma

Yellow Nails

- Causes

Bronchitis, diabetes, arthritis, hyperthyroidism and lung diseases

Red Nailbed

- Cause

Heart disease

Pale Nailbed

- Cause

Anemia

Argyria (slate gray or blue discoloration of the nailplates)

- Causes

Poisoning due to ingestion of silver or silver salts. Colloidal silver dietary supplements marketed for patients with the following diseases: cancer, aids, diabetes, and herpes. Silver amalgam may be used in surgical and dental procedures.

- Treatment

Selenium, sulfur products and 4 percent hydroquinone treatment

Yellow Nail Syndrome

- Causes

Lymphatic system disease may cause discoloration and thickening of the nailplates. As well as, lymphedema in the legs and feet, and fluid in the lungs.

Subungual Hematoma

Subungual hematoma is blood beneath the nailplate. The blood may either be dried or fresh based on when the trauma occurred.

- Causes

Hematoma of the nailbed can be due to an active lifestyle, narrow toe box or trauma.

- Signs and symptoms

A subungual hematoma can be painful due to an increase in pressure beneath the nailplate.

- Treatment

If the hematoma is due to a recent injury and the blood is bright red and liquefied the podiatrist may use a sterile instrument to drill a small hole in the nailplate to drain the blood. Proper wound care will be needed. If the hematoma is the result of an old injury and the blood is dried, the nailplate will probably be loose and the podiatrist will debride the toenail and clean the nailbed with hydrogen peroxide. The nailplate will regrow.

- Prevention

Preventing the causative factors is important. Proper shoe gear with a wide toe box is recommended. Wearing shoe gear when performing certain tasks can help avoid injury to the toes and nailplates.

Onychocryptosis (Ingrown toenail) (picture 4)

Onychocryptosis is an ingrown toenail on the medial or lateral border of the nailplate.

13

- Causes

There are many causes of onychocryptosis such as hereditary factors, trauma, improper nail trimming, and shoe gear.

- Signs and symptoms

An onychocryptotic nail will begin with mild pain at the offending nail border. As time progresses the pain will increase, and signs of edema (swelling), redness, drainage, warmth and peeling of the skin fold may occur.

- Treatment

A podiatrist will debride the offending nail border. Sometimes a local anesthetic is used if the area is painful and inflamed. If the entire nail border is removed this is called a partial nail avulsion. Prior to the partial nail avulsion the entire toe needs to be anesthetized. A chemical or a laser is used to kill the cells that cause the nail to grow. This procedure is done to try and avoid subsequent ingrown toenails. Proper wound care will be needed.

- Prevention

Proper nail debridement is important to prevent an ingrown toenail. Toenails should always be cut straight across and never into the corners. If the nail plate has a natural curvature or if the corner of the nail is beginning to be painful a podiatrist can debride the toenails and avoid the progression of an ingrown toenail.

Proper shoe gear with a wide toe box is also recommended to avoid pressure on the sides of the toenails.

Paronychia (picture 4)

Paronychia is an infection of the nail fold surrounding the nailplate. Usually paronychia occurs due to an ingrown toenail.

- Causes

Bacteria, fungi or viruses

- Signs and symptoms

The offending nailfold will be painful, especially with pressure from shoe gear and socks. Redness, edema, temperature change and drainage may all be present on the offending nailfold. The nail may change shape and nail loss may result.

- Treatment

A podiatrist will debride the offending nail border, usually using a local anesthetic. Proper wound care will be needed. Oral antibiotics may need to be prescribed. The patient will be instructed on daily wound care and a surgical shoe may be necessary. If paronychia is the result of chronic ingrown toenails the podiatrist may suggest a partial nail avulsion to avoid subsequent nail problems. A chemical or laser will be used to kill the cells that make the nail grow.

Koilonychia (concave nails, spoon shaped nails) (picture 5)

The nailplate is concave and resembles the shape of a spoon. If a drop of water is placed on the nailplate it will stay in place and not roll off the nail. In adults, concave nails are usually related to a systemic disorder, however in infants concave nails are normal.

- Causes

Some causes of koilonychia are iron defiency anemia, trauma, Raynaud's disease, syphilis, diabetes and thyroid disorders.

- Signs and symptoms

Concave nails will appear brittle with rounded edges.

- Treatment

The disease causing the concave nails needs to be treated once under control the nails should return to normal.

- Reflexology

Working the reflex zones that relate to the systemic disorder may aid in symptomatology of the disease process.

Beau Lines (picture 6)

Beau lines are white, linear, horizontal ridges on the nailplate. Thinning of the nailplate may be present.

- Causes

Beau lines may be due to trauma, malnutrition, high fever, shock, myocardial infarction (heart attack), chemotherapy and any disease process that causes severe interruption of protein formation.

- Treatment

The disease process that is causing beau lines needs to be treated. Once under control the nails should return to normal.

- Reflexology

Working the reflex zones that relate to the systemic disorder may aid in symptomatology of the disease process.

Clubbed Nails (picture 7)

Clubbed nails change the appearance of the nails and the digits.

- Causes

Clubbed nails occur in disorders that affect the oxygen level in the blood.

Clubbed nails can be seen in children with abnormal heart anatomy or heart disease.

In adults, clubbed nails are a symptom of lung disease including cancer or infection. Cardiac and gastrointestinal disease can also cause clubbed nails.

Unilateral clubbed nails are defined as clubbing on either one hand or one foot. The causes of unilateral clubbing are injury, tumors, sarcoidosis (inflammatory disease affecting any interior or exterior body part) or hyperthroidism.

- Signs and symptoms

The distal aspect of the digits become rounded and resembles a bulb. The nailbed becomes spongy which causes the nailplate to become elevated from the nailbed. The nailplate may be curved up to 180 degrees. The nailplate resembles the back of a spoon.

- Treatment

The cause of the disease needs to be treated and the affected digits and nailplates will return to normal.

- Reflexology

Working the reflex zones that relate to the systemic disorder may aid in symptomatology of the disease process.

Psoriasis (picture 8)

Psoriasis is an increase in the cell cycle of epidermal cells. The normal cell cycle is three to four weeks; psoriasis increases the cell cycle to four days. Nail changes occur in 50 percent of individuals with psoriasis.

- Signs and symptoms

Pitting and splitting of the nailplate from the nailbed occurs, eventually leading to the destruction of the nailplate. Nails may also become thick, yellow and crumbly, mimicking onychomycosis. A thorough patient history and laboratory analysis of the nailplate will aid in diagnosis of the condition.

- Treatment

Treatment of systemic psoriasis needs to be addressed before nail changes will resolve.

- Reflexology

Working the reflex zones which correspond to psoriasis may help with the systemic disease process. The reflex zones I concentrate on for psoriasis are the solar plexus, kidney, pituitary, adrenal, thyroid and parathyroid glands.

Splinter Hemorrhages

- Causes

Splinter hemorrhages are caused by microscopic clots that damage the small capillaries underneath the nail plate. They are associated with bacterial and fungal endocarditis, vasculitis and microemboli. Acute trauma or repetitive stress can cause splinter hemorrhages that will grow out distally as the nailplate grows. Athletes may tend to have splinter hemorrhages due to microtrauma to their toenails.

- Signs and symptoms

Splinter hemorrhages are brown or red lesions that run longitudinally beneath the nailplate. Splinter hemorrhages are not painful.

- Treatment

If a client presents with splinter hemorrhages and is unaware of them send them to their medical doctor. A systemic problem needs to be ruled out.

Nail polish

Chronic exposure to nail polish can produce brittle nails that tend to peel at the edges.

Periungual Warts (picture 9)

Warts that are found around the fingernail may grow under

the fingernail. Warts under the fingernail may change the shape of the nail. Warts are a virus and can be contagious.

- Treatment

If the wart is beneath the nailplate surgery may be needed to remove the nailplate. The wart can be removed by laser, freezing or chemicals.

Lichen Planus (picture 10)

A viral infection can cause lichen planus. Lichen planus is an abnormal immune reaction, in which the inflammatory cells mistake the skin cells for foreign cells and attack them.

- Signs and symptoms

Lichen planus can cause shedding or destruction of the nailplate. There is usually no pain involved.

- Treatment

Lichen planus is treated with steroids and phototherapy.

White Spots

White spots on the nailplate are common and usually grow out. They are usually due to trauma to the base of the nail.

Hutchinson's Sign

Hutchinson's sign is a brown or black pigmentation on the nailbed, nailplate, nailfolds and cuticle.

- Cause

Hutchinson's sign can be caused by a subungual melanoma that usually affects the hallux (big toe). Hutchinson's sign most commonly affects men age 60 and older.

- Treatment

The treatment for subungual melanoma is surgical excision of the tumor.

Muehrcke's Lines

The affected nailplate will present with two white transverse lines. When pressure is applied to the distal aspect of the digit the lines will disappear, when the pressure is released the lines will reappear.

- Causes

Muehrcke's lines may be caused by hypoalbuminemia. Hypoalbuminemia is a decrease in albumin in the body. Albumin is a protein that is responsible for transporting bilirubin, fatty acids, metals, ions, hormones and exogenous drugs.

Onychotillomania

Onychotillomania is a compulsive habit of picking the nails and cuticles. This disorder is seen most often in people with anorexia nervosa and bulimia.

Chromonychia

Chromonychia is a brown stain on the nailplate due to coffee, nicotine, tar and formaldehyde.

CHAPTER 3

OSSEOUS PATHOLOGY

OSSEOUS PATHOLOGY

Bunion (Hallux Abducto Valgus) (picture 11)

A bunion deformity is an enlargement of bone or tissue around the joint. The first metatarsalphalangeal joint (joint of the big toe) is affected. The toe bends laterally (towards the other toes) and the first metatarsal bone moves medially (away from the other toes) causing the deformity in the joint.

- Causes

A bunion deformity may be due to hereditary factors, shoe gear or systemic conditions such as arthritis.

- Signs and symptoms

A bunion deformity usually will present with pain around the first metatarsalphalangeal joint. As the deformity progresses edema, increased pain, tenderness, redness and a callous may develop.

Sometimes the second digit can become deformed and overlap the big toe this can be painful and make shoes uncomfortable. Hammertoes can also occur in the other digits due to pressure from the big toe. Decreased motion in the first metatarsalphalangeal joint is common and can cause an abnormal gait (walk). An abnormal gait can lead to knee, hip and back pain.

- Treatment

A podiatrist will try and accommodate a bunion deformity with shoe gear, pads and orthotics. If problems persist anti-inflammatory medication, corticosteroid injections and/or surgery may be suggested.

- Reflexology

On patients that have a bunion deformity I work the lung reflex on the plantar aspect of the foot. I have found a correlation between lung problems and symptomatic bunion deformities. I also work directly on the bunion deformity to help reduce inflammation around the offending joint.

Tailor's Bunion

Similar to the bunion of the hallux this bunion occurs in the fifth digit (small toe). With a tailor's bunion the fifth metatarsal bone shifts laterally and the fifth metatarsalphalangeal joint is affected.

- Causes

A tailor's bunion may be due to hereditary factors, flatfeet, shoe gear with a narrow toe box or inflammatory diseases such as arthritis.

- Signs and symptoms

A tailor's bunion may cause pain especially if the bony

prominence rubs against the shoe gear. As time progresses, increased pain, redness, edema and a callous may develop.

- Treatment

A podiatrist will try and accommodate the deformity with pads, orthotics and proper shoe gear. Shoe gear is very important with bone deformities. It is important to avoid shoes with a lot of stitching. Any stitching on the inside of the shoe may rub on the protruding bone and cause pain, blisters and ulcerations (sores). A shoe with a wide toe box will be able to accommodate bone deformities such as a bunion or hammertoe. If the pain progresses the podiatrist may prescribe anti-inflammatory medication, corticosteroid injections or suggest surgery to correct the bone deformity.

- Reflexology

I suggest working on the shoulder reflex and directly on the fifth metatarsalphalangeal joint area to help reduce inflammation around the joint and soft tissues. Only apply as much pressure as the patient can tolerate. A joint may be sensitive when it is inflamed.

Hammertoe (picture 12)

A hammertoe is a digit that is deformed at the proximal-interphalangeal joint (middle joint). The toe may be flexible with movement at the joint or rigid with no movement at the joint. The second digit is most often affected.

- Causes

Hammertoes can be due to hereditary factors, shoe gear, muscle imbalance or arthritis.

- Signs and symptoms

Hammertoes can be painful due to the bony prominence rubbing on the shoe gear that causes friction. Friction between the bone and the shoe will cause a corn to develop over the affected area. If friction continues the corn may ulcerate (sore) and a wound will develop.

- Treatment

If the area is inflamed anti-inflammatory medication or a corticosteroid injection may be prescribed. Shoe gear should be evaluated to insure the toe box is large enough to accommodate the deformed digit. The podiatrist may recommend orthotics. Padding the area with moleskin to take pressure off the corn may help. Never use medicated corn and callous pads to remove the corn; the pads can burn the skin and lead to ulcerations. Surgery is sometimes recommended to correct a hammertoe.

- Prevention

Proper shoe gear with a wide toe box and felt or foam pads to protect bony prominences from friction.

- Reflexology

In my practice I have found a correlation between hammertoes and sinus problems. I have had success with flexible hammertoes by working directly on the hammertoe to help reduce inflammation. I work on the following reflexes for sinus problems: sinuses, ileocecal valve, adrenal and pituitary glands.

Mallot toe (picture 12)

A mallot toe is a deformity at the distal interphalangeal joint of the digit (joint at the end of the toe). The affected joint at the tip of the toe is turned down against the shoe and is not able to straighten.

- Causes

A mallot toe can be due to hereditary factors, muscle imbalance, shoe gear or arthritis.

- Signs and symptoms

Weight bearing activities cause pressure on the area, leading to the development of a callous at the tip of the mallot toe. With continued pressure the callous can ulcerate and become infected. Pain may accompany this deformity due to pressure on the distal aspect of the digit.

- Treatment

A podiatrist needs to debride a callous with a scalpel blade.

Proper shoe gear with a wide toe box is needed. If the area becomes ulcerated or an infection occurs appropriate antibiotics and wound care is necessary. Surgery may be needed if the deformity is problematic. The distal aspect of the digit where the corn is located is a difficult area to pad.

- Prevention

Proper shoe gear with a wide toe box is recommended.

- Reflexology

I work directly on the affected digit to help decrease inflammation. If there is an ulcer or infection do not work directly on the area. The location of the mallot toe deformity correlates with the brain reflex.

Claw toe (picture 12)

A claw toe is a combination of a hammertoe and a mallot toe. The claw toe deformity affects both the middle and distal (end) joints of the toe. Claw toes can occur in any toe, except the hallux.

- Causes

A claw toe may be due to hereditary factors, muscle imbalance or arthritis.

- Signs and symptoms

A flexible claw toe means the toe can be straightened

30

manually. With a rigid claw toe the toe cannot be manually straightened and movement of the toe is limited. The toe can become painful. Corns and callouses may develop and with constant pressure they can ulcerate and become infected.

- Treatment

Proper shoe gear is needed to accommodate deformities. Padding is recommended. Surgery is an option.

- Prevention

Proper shoe gear with a wide toe box is recommended. Pad bony prominences using felt or foam pads.

- Reflexology

I work directly on the affected digit to help decrease inflammation. If an ulceration or infection is present reflexology is not recommended. The claw toe deformity corresponds with the brain and sinus reflexes.

Metatarsalgia

Metatarsalgia is pain on the plantar (bottom) aspect of the foot, under the metatarasal heads (ball of foot).

- Causes

Metatarsalgia can be due to foot structure, shoes with a narrow toe box, or loss of the plantar fat pad under the ball of the foot, a common occurrence during the aging process.

- Signs and symptoms

Pain occurs on the bottom of the foot and callouses form under the metatarsal heads due to weight bearing pressure.

- Treatment

The cause of metatarsalgia has to be determined and treated. Proper shoe gear is important. A shoe with a wide toe box will give the digits and metatarsals more space. High heels and backless shoes will cause more pressure on the ball of the foot and cause pain and symptomatology. Padding the ball of the foot will help relieve pressure on the metatarsal heads and decrease callous formation.

- Prevention

Proper shoe gear with a wide toe box is recommended. Moleskin or felt to pad the ball of the foot may help.

- Reflexology

I work on the ball of the foot to help ease the pain and inflammation. The reflex zones in this area are the lung and diaphragm reflexes.

Sesamoiditis

The sesamoids are two small bones under the hallux that are connected to the flexor hallucis longus muscle.

The sesamoid bones help with weight bearing and elevate the hallux. Sometimes these bones can fracture or the tendon they are connected to can become inflamed and painful.

- Causes

Fracture or sesamoiditis (inflammation of the tendon surrounding the bones) can be due to excessive pressure on the ball of the foot especially under the hallux. Commonly diagnosed in ballet dancers, runners and baseball catchers.

- Signs and symptoms

With sesamoiditis the pain is gradual and edema may be present. If the sesamoid bone is fractured the area can be extremely painful upon weight bearing due to the location of the sesamoid bones.

- Treatment

Treatment for sesamoiditis includes x-rays, modification of activity so the patient is not on the ball of their foot, anti-inflammatory medication, felt pads and rest.

Treatment for a sesamoid fracture includes x-rays, a brace or cast to stabilize the area, anti-inflammatory medication and possibly surgery.

- Prevention

Sport specific shoes with adequate support.

- Reflexology

If the area were fractured I would not do reflexology directly on the sesamoid bone. If sesamoiditis is the diagnosis reflexology can be performed only to the patient's tolerance level.

Haglund's Deformity

Haglund's deformity is a painful bump on the back of the heel where the achilles tendon attaches to the heel bone.

- Causes

Haglund's deformity can be due to hereditary factors, weight gain, injury to the area or improper shoe gear.

- Signs and symptoms

The patient may experience pain in the back of the heel, redness, edema and bursitis (fluid filled sack behind the heel and tendon which becomes inflamed).

- Treatment

A podiatrist may prescribe orthotics and or anti-inflammatory medication. Ice on the area may help reduce the inflammation, especially after an activity. Surgery to remove the bump on the heel may be an option.

- Prevention

Supportive shoes that do not irritate the back of the heel are recommended. Stitching on the inside of the shoe in the heel area should be avoided.

- Reflexology

Reflexology treatments can help reduce inflammation in the heel area where the haglund's deformity is located. If the area does not have a blister or sore, I work directly on the deformity using the appropriate pressure the person can tolerate.

Callouses

A callous (dead skin) is a thick layer of skin over a bony prominence (exostosis).

- Causes

Callouses develop due to pressure between the bone and external forces. External forces can be gravitational forces on a bony prominence or shoe gear that rubs on a bony prominence. The body builds a callous over the bony prominence to protect the area, however overtime the callous can break down and ulcerate or blister.

- Signs and symptoms

The build up of a callous is usually on the plantar aspect of the foot or on an area where the shoe rubs on a bony prominence. A callous on the back of the heel can become a heel fissure (crack or crevice). A callous may become painful.

- Treatment

The cause of the callous needs to be identified and treated. A callous on the plantar aspect of the ball of the foot is usually due to a metatarsal head that is plantarflexed and receives more pressure from gravitational forces when walking then the other metatarsals. In this case the callous can be debrided with a scalpel blade. However, if the plantarflexed metatarsal is not corrected, in a few weeks to months the callous may return. Padding the callous with felt or moleskin will help delay its growth rate. Never use medicated corn and callous remover pads; they tend to burn the dead and healthy skin. Surgery on the bone that has an exostosis is an option. Heel fissures can be difficult to treat due to constant friction on the heel, usually from shoe gear. A podiatrist will debride the thick skin and a lubricating cream should be applied on a regular basis to help soften the area. If the area is infected antibiotic cream is used and proper cleansing of the area is required.

- Prevention

Proper shoe gear to accommodate the foot structure is important for callous development. If a person has a bunion and tends to develop callouses on the plantar and medial aspect of their foot then a shoe with a wide toe box is important. Be careful of stitching on the shoe because any stitching on the outside of the shoe is usually on the inside as well and the bony prominence may rub on the stitching and become calloused and perhaps even ulcerate.

- Reflexology

Depending on the location of the callous, working on the offending bone and directly on the callous will help with inflammation. Pressure should be applied to the patient's tolerance level. If the calloused area has a blister or an infection I do not recommend reflexology.

Heloma Dura

Heloma dura is a hard corn. A corn is a thickening of skin over a bony prominence that receives pressure, usually from shoe gear.

- Causes

Corns are due to the structure of the foot. If a person has a hammertoe the affected joint will be elevated due to the contracted digit. The elevated joint will be under constant pressure when wearing shoes and a corn may develop.

- Signs and symptoms

The build up of dead skin (corn) is the body's method of protection from constant pressure on the offending area. If the hard, dead skin is not debrided and pressure continues the corn will eventually break down and blister or ulcerate. The corn may be painful and inflamed and may also become infected.

- Treatment

A podiatrist will debride the corn. Shoes with a wide toe box are important to accommodate structural deformities. Padding the corn with felt, moleskin or tube foam will help. Never use medicated corn and callous remover pads they tend to burn the dead and healthy skin. Surgery on the bony deformity that is causing the corn may be an option.

- Prevention

Proper shoe gear with a wide toe box will help give the toes enough room. Avoid stitching on the shoes in the toe box area. Stitching on the outside of the shoe means there is stitching on the inside of the shoe that may cause friction between the bony prominence and the shoe.

- Reflexology

If the corn is due to a flexible toe deformity (can manually extend the digit straight), reflexology on the digit can help reduce the deformity and inflammation. With a rigid digit deformity (cannot manually extend the digit straight) reflexology will help with pain and inflammation.

Heloma Molle (picture 13)

A heloma molle is a soft corn between the digits.

- Causes

The bones between the two digits rub together and create friction. In response to the friction the body builds dead skin between the digits. This dead skin remains soft between the two digits.

- Signs and symptoms

The soft corn can become painful, especially if the shoe gear has a narrow toe box that allows the toes to rub together and cause friction, resulting in a heloma molle. Sometimes the heloma molle can become infected.

- Treatment

The shoe gear must provide a wide enough toe box to allow the toes enough room. A narrow toe box will push the toes close together and symptoms will worsen due to constant friction between the digits. Padding the area between the toes is difficult; adhesive does not stick well in a moist environment. Tube foam on one of the offending digits works well although it is bulky in the shoe. A podiatrist will debride the soft corn and treat the infection if one occurs. Surgery may be an option.

- Prevention

Shoe gear with a wide toe box and tube foam is recommended.

- Reflexology

The web spaces (area between the digits) are a difficult area on which to perform reflexology.

Heel Spur Syndrome/Plantar Fascitis (picture 14)

Heel spur syndrome, also known as plantar fascitis, is inflammation due to stress on the plantar aspect of the calcaneous. The origin of the plantar fascia is on the plantar aspect of the calcaneous known as the calcaneal tuberosity.

- Causes

The plantar fascia is a tissue similar to a tendon on the bottom of the foot. The plantar fascia originates at the calcaneous and inserts into the base of the toes. When the plantar fascia is excessively stretched, symptoms of plantar fascitis can occur. Stretching of the plantar fascia causes pulling at the origin of the fascia, the calcaneal tuberosity. Repetitive pulling at the origin of the fascia on the calcaneous causes inflammation and pain. In response to the inflammation the body will produce bone in the area, hence the name heel spur. However it is not the bone, but the pulling at the origin of the plantar fascia which causes pain.

Pulling at the origin of the plantar fascia is caused by pressure on the ball of the foot. This pressure may cause the plantar fascia to be stretched and pulling will occur at the origin of the fascia, on the calcaneal tuberosity. The following are examples of activities that cause pressure on

40

the ball of the foot:

1. Kneeling with the ball of the foot on the ground while the heel is off the ground.

2. Reaching up while keeping the ball of the foot on the ground and the heel off the ground.

3. Riding a bike with toe clips.

4. Working out on a stairmaster and the ball of the foot is touching the pedal but the heel is lifted and not touching the pedal.

5. Downward dog position in yoga is when the heel does not make contact with the ground and the ball of the foot is on the ground.

6. Kickboxing and running. Where the ball of the foot makes contact with the ground but the heel does not.

7. Going up and down steps with the heel off the ground and only the ball of the foot making contact with the step.

8. Climbing a ladder using the ball of the foot.

Shoes that support the heel are important. Avoid backless

shoes, thongs, slippers and going barefoot. This footgear does not support the heel and creates pressure on the ball of the foot, pulling the plantar fascia. Weight gain may cause pressure on the balls of the feet in turn causing heel spur symptoms. Rapid weight gain from pregnancy is a common factor.

- Signs and symptoms

The patient will usually say, "My feet hurt when I first get out of bed in the morning." Pain upon standing after sitting or lying down is the most common complaint. Most people say the pain is similar to a pin sticking in the bottom of their foot. The pain usually causes the patient to change the way they are walking to compensate for the pain. It may also make them stop activity or cause tendonitis in other areas of the foot.

- Treatment

A podiatrist will usually take x-rays. Physical therapy may be recommended and corticosteroid injections may be used. In addition anti-inflammatory medication and orthotics may help. The key to treatment is educating the patient on the causes of heel spur pain and how to avoid plantarflexion of the foot (heel off the ground) in everyday activity. Stretching the achilles tendon is very important since the achilles tendon can become contracted and tight with heel spur syndrome (picture 15). Activities such as yoga and kickboxing do not have to stop; they have to be modified so the heel is never off the ground when the ball of the foot is on the ground. I suggest the patient wear supportive shoes even upon getting out of bed. Make sure a pair of gym shoes are beside the bed. Surgery is needed only 1 percent of the time.

- Prevention

Avoid the causes of heel spur syndrome and always wear supportive shoes.

- Reflexology

Reflexology can be extremely beneficial in heel spur patients. Working the entire plantar aspect of the foot, especially on the heel, can decrease inflammation and pain. Working the achilles tendon area on the posterior aspect of the heel and leg will help with a tight achilles tendon and inflammation. In my medical practice I have had great success with reflexology treatments and patient education. It does not take many treatments to make a difference, however the patient needs to be compliant and modify activity so pressure on the ball of the foot is decreased.

Fractures

A fracture is a break in a bone. A stress fracture is a fracture caused by repetitive trauma to a bone.

- Cause

The most common cause of a fracture is trauma.

- Signs and symptoms

Fractures usually present with pain, edema and bruising.

- Treatment

A podiatrist will usually take an x-ray. A stress fracture may not show on an x-ray immediately. Treatment of a fracture includes immobilization with a cast or a splint. Crutches may be needed. Elevation of the leg is important to help decrease edema. Anti-inflammatory medication will help with edema and pain. Surgery is sometimes needed if the two bones do not align properly. Fractures usually take six to eight weeks to heal.

- Reflexology

Reflexology is not recommended on a fractured site. However, a light reflexology treatment around the fracture site and on the rest of the foot will increase blood flow to the foot and help heal the fracture.

CHAPTER 4

ARTHRITIS

Arthritis

Arthritis is inflammation of a joint. There are many different types of arthritis. DJD (degenerative joint disease), also known as osteoarthritis, is the most common type. Other types of arthritis are rheumatoid, gouty, septic and psoriatic.

DJD (Degenerative Joint Disease or Osteoarthritis)

- Causes

Degenerative joint disease is most commonly due to trauma to a joint, usually from long term overuse. The two sides of bone forming the joint are covered with cartilage. When the cartilage is destroyed from long term overuse the bones begin to rub together causing osteoarthritis. The bone will form osteophytes due to the pressure. Osteophytes are bone spurs around the joint.

- Signs and symptoms

Affected joints will be painful only during activity, edema and stiffness will follow.

- Treatment

X-rays are important to evaluate the joint structure. Anti-inflammatory medication may help. Physical therapy, padding of affected joints and shoe gear may help.

- Reflexology

I recommend working on patients with DJD; it helps with the pain and inflammation. However, if the joint is painful work lightly on affected areas. Other reflexes to work for arthritis include the solar plexus, kidneys, adrenal, pituitary, thyroid and parathyroid glands.

Rheumatoid Arthritis

Rheumatoid arthritis is an inflammatory disease that destroys the affected joints.

- Causes

The cause of rheumatoid arthritis is not entirely understood; it is believed that the body attacks a specific antibody in the blood that results in inflammation.

- Signs and symptoms

According to the American Rheumatism Association, four of the seven symptoms stated below have to exist before rheumatoid arthritis can be diagnosed. The symptoms are as follows:

> 1. Morning stiffness around the joints lasting at least one hour before improvement. The morning stiffness has to be continuous for six weeks minimum.

2. Arthritis of at least three or more joints for six weeks minimum.

3. Arthritis of joints in the hand for six weeks minimum.

4. Symmetrically arthritis, the same joints are affected on both sides of the body for a minimum of six weeks.

5. Rheumatoid nodules (visible bumps on joint) observed.

6. Positive blood test for serum rheumatoid factor.

7. Changes in the affected joints noticeable on x-ray.

- Treatment

A podiatrist will encourage the patient to exercise and maintain flexibility and strength. Orthotics or custom molded shoes may help especially if the foot has changed shape due to joint deformities. Anti-inflammatory medication may also help with inflammation of the joint. A destroyed joint may be replaced by an implant.

- Prevention

Exercise may decrease the severity of the condition.

- Reflexology

In my practice, I see many people with rheumatoid arthritis. Reflexology treatments help with the inflammation and pain, especially if the treatments are consistent. The following are the reflexes I concentrate on for arthritis: solar plexus, kidneys, thyroid, parathyroid, adrenal and pituitary glands

Gouty Arthritis

Gouty arthritis results from an accumulation of uric acid crystals.

- Causes

Foods that contain a high purine level such as, liver, kidneys, shellfish and sardines, can cause gout. Consuming these foods causes the body to produce too much uric acid too quickly. Another cause of gout is when the body cannot process and eliminate uric acid fast enough. This can be due to low dose aspirin therapy, thiazide diuretics, excessive drinking or surgery. The result is hyperuricemia (increased uric acid) in the blood. The uric acid forms uric crystals and the crystals form gouty tophi.

- Signs and symptoms

Gouty arthritis can cause severe pain, edema, redness, heat and stiffness of the affected joint. Gout is common in the first metatarsalphalangeal joint and is called Podagra.

- Treatment

A doctor will order a blood test to check the levels of uric acid in the body. Anti-inflammatory medication and sometimes an injection of medication is needed.

- Prevention

Eliminate high purine foods in the diet and decrease alcohol consumption.

- Reflexology

I would not recommend working on a patient with an acute attack of gout. However, if someone has a history of gout but they are not symptomatic, I will work directly on a non-symptomatic gouty joint. According to a patient, I have prevented a gouty attack from occurring. I also work on the following reflexes: kidneys, lymph nodes and pituitary gland.

Septic Arthritis

Septic arthritis is due to an infection in the blood.

- Causes

Many types of infection can cause inflammation and thickening of the synovial joint fluid. The increase in fluid can cause destruction of cartilage and destroy the joint surface. Gonorrhea is a common infection that causes septic arthritis.

- Signs and symptoms

Septic arthritis can cause pain in one or more joints. The infection will cause many more symptoms throughout the body.

- Treatment

The doctor will take x-rays to evaluate the joints. Anti-inflammatory medication may be prescribed to reduce inflammation. Aspiration of the joint will help identify the cause of the infection and aid in choosing the proper antibiotic for treatment.

- Prevention

In septic arthritis immediate diagnosis is important to decrease joint destruction.

- Reflexology

I would not recommend working on a patient with septic arthritis until the infection is entirely gone.

51

Psoriatic Arthritis (picture 16)

Psoriatic arthritis presents with skin lesions and pitting of the nailplates.

- Causes

The cause of psoriatic arthritis is unknown; it could be due to genetics, bacterial or a viral organism.

- Signs and symptoms

Affected joints are painful and are usually unilateral. An entire toe or digit on a foot can be affected and will look like a "sausage digit". Skin lesions that look like white patches are located most often on elbows, shins, and ankles. Pitting of the nailplates is usually present. The joints can erode and become so damaged they have an opera glass appearance or a pencil in cup appearance.

- Treatment

Exercise is important to decrease stiffness and inflammation of the affected joint. Anti-inflammatory medication may be prescribed to help decrease inflammation. If the joint is destroyed an implant may be necessary or the joint may need to be fused.

- Reflexology

I have a patient who has psoriatic arthritis in his hands. His metacarpal and phalangeal bones in his hands are pencil thin. Due to the psoriatic arthritis the joint is pencil thin at one end and wide like the base of a cup at the adjacent end of the joint. I work directly on the affected digit including the joint to decrease pain and inflammation. I also work on the following reflexes for psoriasis: the solar plexus, kidney, adrenal, pituitary, thyroid and parathyroid glands.

Neuropathic Osteoarthropathy (Charcot Joint) (picture 17)

Neuropathic osteoarthropathy is a rapidly progressive degenerative arthritis resulting from damaged nerves.

- Causes

When a patient suffers from neuropathy the blood vessels become lax and blood flow increases to the feet due to gravitational forces. The increased blood flow demineralizes and weakens the bone, allowing microfractures to begin. The patient now has neuropathy and cannot feel pain. As the patient continues to bear weight microfractures continue. The bone lays down new bone in response to the fractures, which is called reconstruction. The pattern of microfractures and reconstruction continues and the foot becomes structurally deformed. Some causes of neuropathy are: diabetes, alcoholism, leprosy and syphilis.

- Signs and symptoms

For neuropathic osteoarthropathy to occur neuropathy has to be present. The foot becomes structurally deformed and the patient usually sees a doctor when their talus bone has rotated medially and plantarly and they are literally walking on the head of their talus bone. This can lead to callous formation and eventually an ulceration (picture 18). For the diabetic patient their sugar is most likely elevated and has been for sometime.

- Treatment

The doctor will take x-rays to view the joint structure. Custom molded shoes are recommended especially if the patient is walking on their talus bone. If an ulceration is present, proper wound care is needed by a physician.

- Prevention

Preventing the cause of neuropathy is the key to preventing the debilitating joint damage. If neuropathy is from diabetes, blood sugar needs to be under control. If neuropathy is from alcoholism proper counseling and treatment may be needed. It is easier to prevent the causes of Charcot Joint then to deal with a structurally deformed foot and chronic ulcerations.

- Reflexology

I have worked on many patients with Charcot Joint due to diabetes. I work directly on the affected joints to decrease inflammation, tendonitis and muscle strain. I do not recommend working directly on an ulceration. Reflexology can be done on the foot, excluding the ulcer, to increase blood flow. An increase in blood flow may also increase the efficacy of the antibiotic, allowing the ulceration to heal faster.

CHAPTER 5

ARCHES

Arches

Pediatric Flatfoot

Flatfoot means a decreased arch on the inside border of the foot when weight bearing.

- Causes

Children are born with flexible flatfoot. When a child stands, the arch on the inside border of the foot goes flat. Most children outgrow flexible flatfoot. As the child grows their lax ligaments and muscles become stronger and their bones increase in size. From age five and up the flexible flatfoot continually decreases and an arch is established.

- Signs and symptoms

Usually pediatric flatfoot corrects itself overtime; it is not painful and does not interfere with walking or sports. If the flatfoot deformity does not correct by adolescence, the child may complain of aching pain on the bottom of their foot.

- Treatment

If the child has non-symptomatic mild flatfoot deformity treatment is not necessary. The child should be seen for yearly evaluations by a podiatrist. If the child has a symptomatic flatfoot deformity then treatment usually begins with shoe gear. Most podiatrists will recommend orthotics and supportive shoes such as high tops. Daily stretches for the achilles tendon are important since many people with flatfoot have tight heel cords. If the child's flatfoot deformity is severe and does not improve with any of the above treatments foot surgery may be an option.

- Reflexology

Reflexology on the child will help with the pain related to the flatfoot deformity. Work directly on the plantar aspect (bottom) of the foot especially along the length of the abductor hallucis muscle and plantar fascia.

Adult Flatfoot

Adult flatfoot deformity is a decreased arch upon weight bearing.

- Causes

Adult flatfoot deformity can be due to hereditary factors, bone structure, neuromuscular disorders or limb length differences. Acquired causes of adult flatfoot include systemic diseases such as: diabetes, obesity, arthritis, trauma or posterior tibial tendon dysfunction.

Posterior tibial tendon dysfunction is the most common acquired cause of flatfoot deformity. The posterior tibial tendon functions to invert the foot (form an arch). If the tendon is dysfunctional the foot will evert (become flat). The posterior tibial tendon can become dysfunctional due to degenerative disease and trauma.

- Signs and symptoms

The patient may experience pain in the heel and/or arch. The knees, hips and back may also become painful. Excessive pronation may result in joint instability which may cause bone deformities such as bunions, hammertoes and overlapping digits.

- Treatment

There is a wide range of treatments for flatfoot due to the different causes of flatfoot deformity. Treatment can be conservative and include rest, immobilization, anti-inflammatory medication, physical therapy, orthotics or foot and ankle braces.

If the flatfoot is due to posterior tibial tendon dysfunction the cause of the tendon dysfunction needs to be addressed. Surgery may be an option.

- Reflexology

Reflexology treatments on flatfoot deformity are beneficial for reducing pain and inflammation. I work on the plantar aspect of the foot and arch area. If the patient has a posterior tibial tendon rupture I do not recommend reflexology. If the flatfoot deformity is due to a systemic disease, I suggest working on the reflexes that correspond to that disease process.

Cavus foot

A cavus foot is a foot with a high arch.

- Causes

High arches can be due to hereditary factors and muscle imbalance in the feet, as well as, neurological disease or muscle diseases such as spina bifida and muscular dystrophy.

Muscle imbalance causes the plantar fascia and plantar ligaments in the foot to become tight, which results in the formation of a high arch.

- Signs and symptoms

High arches decrease the ability of the foot to absorb shock when weight bearing. Pain may occur in the knees, hip, back, heel and ball of foot. Increased pressure on the ball of the foot is common with a cavus foot. This can lead to metatarsalgia, callouses and tendon imbalances which can cause tight tendons and digital deformities such as hammertoes.

- Treatment

Treatment will depend on the cause of the cavus foot. Sometimes a shock absorbing orthotic can help reduce the symptoms. Surgery may also be an option.

- Reflexology

I have an 80-year-old patient with a hereditary cavus foot deformity. Her symptoms include plantar callouses on the ball of her feet, tight tendons on the dorsal (top) aspect of her feet and muscle cramps in her feet. The extensor digitorum tendons on the top of her feet are so tight they bow and stick out, especially when she plantarflexs her feet. The tight extensor digitorum tendons are compressing the superficial peroneal nerve that is on the top of the foot beneath the extensor digitorum tendons. I have worked with the patient to relax her feet, especially when she is lying or sitting down. Reflexology treatments have been very successful in decreasing the inflammation and relaxing the extensor tendons that compress the superficial peroneal nerve. I have used felt to pad the plantar aspect of her shoes to try and relieve the pressure on the balls of her feet.

CHAPTER 6

SOFT TISSUE PATHOLOGY

<u>Soft Tissue Pathology</u>

<u>Tinea Pedis</u>

Tinea pedis is a fungal infection of the skin.

- Causes

Tinea pedis is caused by fungus that can survive and grow on our skin. Fungi like a moist, hot, dark environment, making our feet desirable for fungus infections. People who are on antibiotics, immunosuppressive drugs, steroids or chemotherapy tend to have a greater risk for developing tinea pedis. Individuals suffering from diseases that compromise the immune system, such as diabetes and HIV, are prone to tinea pedis.

- Signs and symptoms

There are 3 forms of tinea pedis:

> 1. Moccasin type- This form usually affects the entire plantar aspect of the foot. The foot will itch and appear slightly red in color with white, scaly tissue in the skin folds. Hyperkeratosis (increased skin) can build up on weight bearing areas of the feet such as the heel. This form is usually chronic.

> 2. Acute vesicular- This form presents as small blisters on the plantar and/or dorsal aspect of the foot. The blisters will itch and

may become larger (bullae). This form usually has a rapid onset.

3. Interdigital- This type of tinea pedis presents in the webspaces (between the toes). It can present either dry, scaly or moist and fissures may develop.

- Treatment

Application of antifungal cream, lotion or powder to the affected area twice daily may treat the fungus. Antifungal powder should be used between the toes to keep the area dry. Oral antifungal medication is an option. Only wear white socks and change socks several times during the day. Spray shoes with Lysol in the evening and let them air out. It is important to dry the feet completely after bathing or swimming, especially between the toes.

- Prevention

Dry both feet and between toes completely after bathing or swimming. Wear sandals in public locker rooms. If your feet tend to perspire alot wear white socks and change them several times daily. Spray shoes with Lysol in the evening. Use a stick deodorant on the bottom of the feet to decrease perspiration.

- Reflexology

Tinea pedis is contagious, especially if the person touching it has a break in their skin. I have a patient whose chief complaint was a sore back and itching on the medial aspect of her foot corresponding to the spinal reflex. The rash on the medial aspect of her foot looked just like tinea pedis. The patient stated the itching woke her up in the middle of the night. She tried every antifungal cream, as well as the oral antifungal medication, and nothing helped. We then talked about the back pain due to carrying her two- year - old on her hip. During her treatment I worked on her spinal reflex intensely. When she returned in three days for her next treatment, I asked her how her back pain was. She stated, " I have not had pain in three days and wait until you see my feet." I looked at her feet and the rash that looked just like tinea pedis was entirely gone. Again, I was amazed at the power of reflexology. The rash was not a fungus infection. It was a rash along the spinal reflex in response to her back pain.

Porokeratosis

A porokeratosis is a plugged sweat gland.

- Cause

The cause of a porokeratosis is due to an obstructed glandular duct.

- Signs and symptoms

Patients will often say, "It feels like I am walking on a stone." Pain upon weight bearing is common.

- Treatment

A podiatrist will debride the porokeratosis. Overtime the porokeratosis will grow back and debridement will be needed. Debridement is noninvasive and is not painful.

Blisters

A blister is a fluid filled lesion.

- Cause

Blisters are caused by friction usually due to a bony prominence rubbing on shoe gear.

- Signs and symptoms

A blister can be painful if the offending shoes are still being worn. A blister is usually filled with clear or bloody fluid (hematoma).

- Treatment

A podiatrist will decompress the blister by using a sterile scalpel blade to release the fluid, followed by antibiotic cream and a bandage. The roof of the blister needs to remain intact to avoid infection. The cause of the blister needs to be identified. If a certain pair of shoes are rubbing on the patient's heel and causing a blister, the shoes should not be worn.

Plantar Wart (Verruca) (picture 19)

Verruca is a wart on the bottom of the foot.

- Cause

The Human Papilloma Virus is the cause of plantar warts.

- Signs and symptoms

Warts are contagious, especially for children and people with a weak immune system. Warts can appear singular or in a cluster called mosaic. A wart will have small pinpoint black dots in the middle of the lesion. These black dots are small blood vessels and are the warts own blood supply. Warts can be painful if the location of the wart has alot of pressure. Warts will bleed upon debridement due to the small blood vessels. Plantar warts are the only warts that grow inward. Black or brown warts may be cancerous.

- Treatments

There are many treatments for warts including:
1. Debridement and application of acid to kill the virus.
2. Cryotherapy to freeze the wart and kill the virus.
3. Laser treatment to kill the virus.

Some holistic methods to treat warts include:
1. Tea tree oil applied on wart daily.
2. Minced, fresh garlic applied on wart daily.
3. Crushed aspirin applied on wart daily.

- Reflexology

Avoid touching warts when giving a reflexology treatment. If you're not sure if a client has a wart look for the black pinpoint dots. Refer the client to a podiatrist for treatment.

Sprains (picture 20)

A sprain is a tearing or stretching of one of the ankle ligaments.

- Causes

A sprain can be caused by a sports injury or trauma. Shoe gear, unlevel ground and loss of balance may also cause sprains.

The most common ankle sprain is an inversion sprain. An inversion sprain is when the foot and ankle turn inward. Three ligaments support the lateral aspect of the ankle. The ligament closest to the digits is usually injured first. This ligament is called the anterior talofibular ligament. It connects the talus bone to the fibular bone. When an ankle sprain occurs, the involved ligament becomes stretched or torn and the ankle swells to prevent further injury.

- Signs and symptoms

Ankle sprains are categorized into three grades.

Grade 1

A grade 1 ankle sprain involves local tenderness and mild edema.

Grade 2

A grade 2 ankle sprain involves edema, bruising and difficulty walking.

Grade 3

A grade 3 ankle sprain involves edema, intense pain, bruising and inability to walk.

- Treatment

Treatment for an ankle sprain varies due to the grade of the sprain. All ankle sprains need RICE (rest, ice, compression and elevation). Never apply heat to an ankle sprain. If a ligament is torn surgery may be indicated.

- Reflexology

I believe reflexology treatments for acute ankle sprains are beneficial. The treatment should be gentle and only to the patient's tolerance level. Reflexology treatments help with the edema and pain. I have found that reflexology right after the ankle injury decreases the healing time of the sprain.

- Proprioception

Ankle sprains damage key nerves that relay information to the brain enabling a person to land properly on their feet when walking. By working on balance a person can retrain these key nerves called proprioceptors so muscles are able to stabilize an ankle if it is about to twist.

Sweaty feet (hyperhidrosis)

Hyperhidrosis is excessive perspiration usually affecting the hands and feet.

- Causes

Hyperhidrosis may be caused by mental or emotional stress, hereditary factors, overactive sweat glands or shoe gear.

- Signs and symptoms

The soles of the feet may be red with moist skin that is cool to the touch. Burning, itching and blister formation may occur. When the feet have an associated odor this is called bromhidrosis, which occurs due to normal bacteria.

- Treatment

Treating the cause of the problem is important. If the cause is due to emotional or mental stress, reflexology on the solar plexus may be useful. The feet should be washed daily with soap and water and dried well to avoid fungal infections. Shoes should be sprayed with Lysol in the evening. White socks should be worn daily and changed periodically during the course of the day. Avoid certain socks and shoes that increase perspiration such as darkly colored socks, pantyhose and vinyl shoes. Foot powders help to reduce friction. Deodorant may reduce perspiration when used on the feet. Caffeine, tea and soda pop can stimulate sweat production and should be avoided.

CHAPTER 7

NERVE PATHOLOGY

Nerve Pathology

Neuroma (picture 21)

A neuroma is an enlarged benign nerve growth usually occurring between the third and fourth digits on the foot. The third web space is the location where the lateral plantar nerve combines with the medial plantar nerve; therefore the nerve diameter is enlarged. When walking the metatarsal heads becomes squeezed together and the nerve becomes compressed causing an enlargement in the nerve and localized pain.

- Causes

A neuroma may be due to abnormal bone structure, shoes with a narrow toe box, shoe gear (high heels), constrictive socks or nylons.

- Signs and symptoms

Neuromas can cause localized dull or sharp pain that can radiate to the distal aspect of the digits. Burning, cramping, tingling or numbness may also develop in the affected foot.

- Treatment

A podiatrist can pad the shoe or foot to relieve the pressure on the affected area. Orthotics may help especially if the orthotic has a built-in pad to relieve pressure from the metatarsal heads when the patient is walking. Avoid high heels which cause the ball of the foot to bear most of the pressure and can create neuroma symptoms. Avoid shoes with a narrow toe box, nylons and tight socks because the metatarsal heads will have less room to splay (spread out). Corticosteroid injections may help with the pain and inflammation temporarily. Surgery may be an option. Even after neuroma surgery symptoms may be evident due to nerve regeneration.

- Prevention

Avoid shoes with a narrow toe box, high heels, tight socks and nylons; they all can cause neuroma symptoms.

- Reflexology

Reflexology is beneficial for the symptoms of a neuroma. The treatment can help with pain, burning, tingling and cramping. It is important to ask the patient about a history of lung problems since the neuroma is located in the lung reflex. Educating the patient about neuromas and proper shoes and socks may help decrease neuroma symptoms.

Dropfoot

Dropfoot is an inability to lift the foot.

- Causes

Dropfoot is due to a reduction in muscle activity or the absence of muscle activity. The major causes of dropfoot are nerve damage, stroke, cerebral palsy and multiple sclerosis. Nerve damage can be due to back surgery, trauma or disease processes.

- Signs and symptoms

The individual with dropfoot cannot control their foot when walking so their foot drops on the ground and their toes drag behind.

- Treatment

If the dropfoot is due to muscle atrophy then increasing the muscle mass through physical therapy may decrease the symptoms. A splint to support the ankle and calf will help with the dropfoot symptoms, however when the splint is removed the dropfoot will be evident.

- Reflexology

In my practice I have had the opportunity to work on a man who had surgery due to a ruptured disc and pinched nerve. After the surgery, the patient had dropfoot of the right foot and he was unable to walk without his brace. He could not play tennis, which he had previously played five to six times a week. This patient began seeing me for reflexology treatments seven months after his surgery. He came twice a week for five weeks. After five weeks he was able to play tennis for one hour without wearing the brace. The patient continues to have reflexology treatments every other week, is able to walk without the brace, and he continues to play tennis. During his treatments I work the entire foot, ankle and lower leg bilaterally.

<u>Peripheral Neuropathy</u>

Peripheral neuropathy is a neurological disorder due to damage of the peripheral nerves.

- Causes

Peripheral nerve damage can be due to systemic diseases or injury to the peripheral nerves. Diabetes, AIDS, uremia, alcoholism and nutritional deficiencies are some systemic diseases that can cause peripheral neuropathy. Fractures, dislocations, lacerations and contusions can all damage the peripheral nerves and lead to peripheral neuropathy.

- Signs and symptoms

Most often peripheral neuropathy will cause a partial or complete loss of sensation. Symptoms may include sensations such as burning, prickling, tickling or tingling.

- Treatment

If a disease is the cause of neuropathy, the treatment is aimed at controlling the disease process. Once the disease is controlled or treated the neuropathy symptoms may decrease or dissipate. If the patient has diabetes, proper sugar control is the most important factor in controlling neuropathy symptoms. If neuropathy is due to trauma then treating the causative agent may decrease symptoms. For example, if a dislocated bone is compressing a nerve and the bone is surgically corrected, the nerve will be released and the neuropathy symptoms may decrease.

- Reflexology

In my practice I have many patients with neuropathy due to injury and diabetes. During the reflexology treatments, I work on the entire foot, however if the neuropathy is due to a systemic disease I also work on the reflexes affected by the disease process. For neuropathy due to an injury I work directly on the injured site including the entire foot. For diabetes, sugar control is very important in the treatment of neuropathy. The neuropathy symptoms can be more severe if the blood sugar is out of control. Educating the patient about diet and exercise is beneficial.

CHAPTER 8

VASCULAR DISEASES

Vascular Diseases

Chronic Venous Insufficiency (picture 22)

Arteries take blood from the heart to the lower extremities while veins take blood from the lower extremities back to the heart. Normal blood flow flows, unidirectionally, from the superficial to the deep veins. The calf muscle helps pump blood back up to the heart. Chronic venous insufficiency is due to diseased veins causing a back flow of blood in the lower legs and feet.

- Causes

Many causes contribute to chronic venous insufficiency such as heart failure, obesity, pregnancy, muscle weakness from paralysis, deep vein thrombosis and venous valve incompetence.

- Signs and symptoms

With long-term chronic venous insufficiency signs and symptoms will become more severe. The disease process will usually begin with mild edema, leg pain, dilated veins, and dry and scaly skin. The skin may begin to feel like leather and itch. If the disease is not controlled, blood will accumulate in the legs and ankles and fluid may begin to leak into the surrounding tissues. Eventually the skin will break down and ulcerate. The skin may have a brown pigmentation due to the accumulation of blood in the legs. This brown discoloration is from the iron in the blood and is called hemosiderin deposits.

79

- Treatment

The cause of the chronic venous insufficiency has to be addressed. Under a doctor's care, edema of the leg has to be controlled by elevating the leg above the heart level or by compression stockings. However, there are contraindications depending on the patient's primary systemic condition. If an ulceration is present proper wound care is advised. If the patient is homebound a doctor can make arrangements for a nurse to visit the patient daily for wound care.

- Reflexology

I have patients with venous insufficiency. Reflexology changes the skin texture and decreases the edema. I do not recommend working on a patient who has deep vein thrombosis (blood clot). Consulting with the patient's medical doctor on the patient's systemic condition is important before starting a reflexology session. If the patient has an ulceration or fluid leakage on their lower legs, I would advise the practitioner to wear gloves and restrict the treatment to the feet only. Apply as much pressure as the patient can tolerate.

Arterial Disease (picture 23)

Arterial disease is a decrease in arterial blood flow to the lower extremity. Remember, arteries bring blood from the heart to the feet and veins bring blood back up to the heart. A decrease in blood flow to the lower extremities due to arterial disease can be chronic or intermittent. Intermittent claudication means blood flow increases and decreases in relationship to demand. If a person is resting, blood flow to the lower extremities will increase and during or after exercise blood flow to the lower extremities will decrease. However, this is the time the blood flow to the lower extremities needs to be increased.

- Causes

There are many causes of arterial disease and intermittent claudication. Smoking is at the top of the list since it narrows the arteries, which will decrease blood flow. Other factors for arterial disease are age, diabetes, high blood pressure, increased cholesterol, plaque due to fatty deposits on arterial walls and hereditary factors.

- Signs and symptoms

The symptoms of arterial disease gradually progress. The earliest most common symptom is pain in the calf muscle when exercising; the pain will decrease and diminish about ten minutes after the patient begins to rest. As the blockage in the arteries increase and the disease becomes more chronic the pain will increase and ulcerations, gangrene and amputation may follow.

- Treatment

The doctor needs to treat the systemic disease that is causing the arterial disease. The patient needs to be responsible for their diet and exercise program. If the arterial disease is chronic and an ulceration is present proper wound care needs to be implemented. Bypass surgery to increase proper blood flow to the affected area may be an option.

- Prevention

Proper diet, exercise, and cessation of smoking are most important.

- Reflexology

Reflexology can increase blood flow to the extremities and help with wound healing. However, the patient has to take responsibility and help themselves through proper diet, exercise and cessation of smoking. If a patient has an ulceration I do not advise reflexology directly on the wound. Apply pressure only to the patient's tolerance level.

Raynaud's Disease

Raynaud's disease is a disorder of the small blood vessels in the digits, causing constriction of the blood vessels. When spasm of the blood vessels occurs there is a decrease of oxygen to the skin causing a blue discoloration of the affected digits. As blood flow and oxygen increase the digits will turn red. As the blood flow normalizes the digits will return to the normal "white" color.

- Causes

Raynaud's disease can occur without any other

contributing factors and is thought to be a reaction to cold or stress. It is associated with other factors such as smoking and certain medications and can be a symptom of many systemic diseases such as scleroderma, lupus, rheumatoid arthritis, hypertension and arteriosclerosis.

- Signs and symptoms

Symptoms usually occur in the digits of the hands and feet and include blue, red and white color changes in one or more digits. The digits may feel numb and tingle.

- Treatment

If Raynaud's disease is due to the cold or stress, addressing those issues is important. Dressing warm with hand and foot warmers or battery-powered mittens may be helpful. If stress is the causative factor it is important to identify the source and work on coping mechanisms. If smoking is the cause cessation is necessary. Medications for blood pressure, migraines, and heart disease may cause Raynaud's symptoms. If Raynaud's is due to a systemic disease treating the condition may decrease the Raynaud's symptoms. Sometimes medications that can dilate the blood vessels and increase blood flow may decrease symptoms.

- Reflexology

Reflexology can help this disease. I have a family history on my mother's side of Raynaud's disease. I, personally, have had Raynaud's for over ten years, my symptoms are not related to any other problem or disease process. My symptoms used to be severe especially during winter. I had to give up many outdoor sports. I used to wear both hand and foot warmers as well as battery operated mittens. Then I began doing reflexology, which allowed my fingers to have constant stimulation on a daily basis. I work on my feet weekly. During the winter I can go with a normal pair of gloves or mittens and my fingers are warm with no symptoms of Raynaud's disease.

<u>Lymphedema (picture 24)</u>

Lymphedema is an abnormal swelling due to an accumulation of lymph fluid (protein rich fluid) in affected areas. Lymph fluid travels through lymph vessels and is filtered through lymph nodes. Lymph fluid, contains white blood cells, and helps our bodies fight infection.
As the fluid enters the lymph nodes bacteria and toxins become trapped and the lymph nodes may swell and become painful. The swelling in lymphedema is due to a blockage in the lymphatic system.

- Causes

Primary lymphedema can be observed at birth or in later years. The cause is unknown. Secondary lymphedema is more common and can be due to surgery, radiation, infection or trauma.

- Signs and symptoms

There are three stages of secondary lymphedema:

84

Stage 1- Edema occurs due to lymph fluid. Elevation of the limb may reduce edema. This edema is called pitting edema. Pitting edema means a thumb pressed on the edematous area will leave an indentation for one or two seconds.

Stage 2- Edema of affected area increases, skin hardens and pitting of tissue decreases.

Stage 3- Limb enlarges due to edema, hard tissue and non-pitting edema. It becomes a breeding ground for bacterial infections. As the lymphedema progresses the function of the affected limb decreases. Progressive skin break down and chronic infections may occur.

- Treatment

If lymphedema is due to an infection, proper antibiotics may be necessary. Under a doctor's supervision, treatment for lymphedema consists of skin care, compression stockings, and exercise and massage to promote lymphatic drainage. Treatment is always based on the cause of the problem.

- Reflexology

I have many patients with lymphedema. The first step is to take a thorough history on the patient and call their

85

physician for information regarding the cause of the lymphedema. Discuss your plan with the doctor and how reflexology can help the patient. If the lymphedema is due to a systemic problem I work on the reflexes pertaining to the systemic problem. I also work on the kidneys, lymph nodes, adrenal and pituitary gland reflexes. I will work on the entire foot, ankle and lower leg as long as there are no open wounds or irritated skin. Apply as much pressure as the patient can tolerate. Keep notes on changes in the patient's affected leg.

CHAPTER 9

DIABETES

Diabetes (picture 25)

Diabetes is a disease in which the body does not produce insulin or cannot properly use insulin. Insulin is a hormone and a protein produced by the pancreas. Most cells in the body have insulin receptor sites on them, which bind the circulating insulin. When a cell can bind insulin it is able to absorb glucose from the bloodstream into the cell. Insulin is needed to convert sugar into energy.

There are two types of diabetes:

> Type 1: Accounting for five to ten percent of all cases, Type 1 diabetes is also known as insulin dependent or juvenile diabetes. In type 1 diabetes the pancreas is unable to produce insulin and sugar remains in the bloodstream while the cells starve for energy. Type 1 usually affects children and young adults.

> Type 2: Also called non-insulin dependent or adult onset diabetes, 90-95 percent of diabetes is type 2. With type 2 diabetes the pancreas may not produce insulin. If insulin is produced the cells may ignore the insulin. This problem is called insulin resistant diabetes. These patients are usually middle age, obese and sedentary.

- Causes

Type 1 diabetes can be hereditary or environmental. Some patients have contracted type 1 diabetes after a flu virus.

Type 2 diabetes can be due to hereditary or environmental factors.

- Signs and symptoms

A person may have diabetes for an extended period of time before they are diagnosed. It is important to have a fasting blood sugar checked at your yearly physical. Some symptoms of diabetes include frequent urination, excessive thirst, excessive hunger, unusual weight loss, fatigue, blurry vision and irritable behavior.

- Treatment

Type 1 diabetics usually require insulin injections or an insulin pump.

Type 2 diabetes can sometimes be controlled by diet and exercise. Most often type 2 diabetics will be prescribed an oral medication and sometimes they may need insulin injections.

The feet are one of the most common areas of the body that are affected by diabetes and high blood sugar levels. Listed below are some foot problems that diabetics may face especially if their sugar is elevated.

1. Peripheral neuropathy- decrease in sensation or tingling in the feet.

2. Decreased circulation- due to diabetes affecting the microcirculation in the feet.

3. Ulcerations- due to the person suffering from neuropathy and not feeling sensations or wounds. If the patient has a foot problem, cannot feel pain, and does not check their feet daily this could lead to an infected wound.

4. Diabetic blisters- small fluid filled blisters on the feet, usually multiple lesions.

5. Charcot joint- destruction of joints due to neuropathy.

Proper sugar control and controlling the effects the blood sugar has on the entire body are the most important factors in diabetes.

- Podiatrist's role

The diabetic patient needs to see their podiatrist on a regular basis for proper trimming of toenails and callouses. The podiatrist will also check the feet for nerve damage and changes in circulation.

- Patient's role

The patient needs to check their feet daily and not go barefoot. Proper hygiene and drying the feet completely after bathing is important. If the patient has neuropathy checking the temperature of the bath water with their hand is important. If they have neuropathy in their hands then using their elbow to check the water temperature is important to avoid burns. Avoid socks with seams. If the patient has neuropathy sometimes a simple seam in the sock can irritate the skin and cause a sore. Proper fitting shoes are important. Shoes with excessive stitching can lead to blisters and infections. Custom molded shoes are a good idea if the patient has foot deformities and joint changes. Never use medicated corn and callous remover pads. These pads burn the dead skin and the surrounding healthy skin which may lead to ulcerations, infections and amputations.

- Reflexology

I have many patients with diabetes and I have found reflexology decreases symptoms of neuropathy and can increase circulation in the feet. If a diabetic has an ulceration I will work on their feet to increase circulation to aid in the healing of the wound. However, I do not advise working directly on the ulceration site. I also work on the following reflex zones for diabetes: spleen, liver, pancreas, pituitary, thyroid, adrenal and parathyroid glands.

Picture 1- Foot bones

Side View of Foot Bones

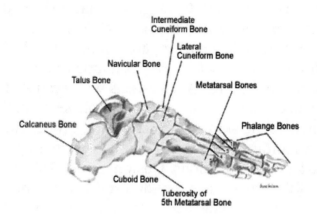

Top View of Foot Bones

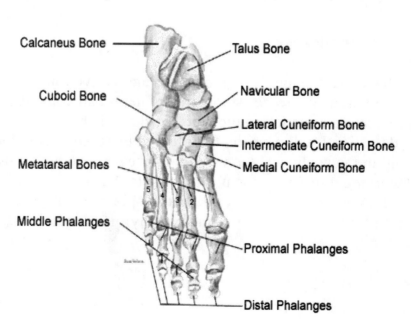

Picture 2- Nail anatomy

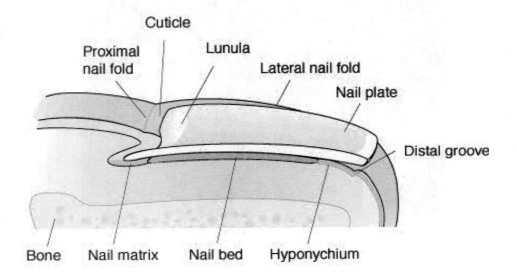

Cuticle
Proximal nail fold
Lunula
Lateral nail fold
Nail plate
Distal groove
Bone
Nail matrix
Nail bed
Hyponychium

Picture 3- Onychomycosis

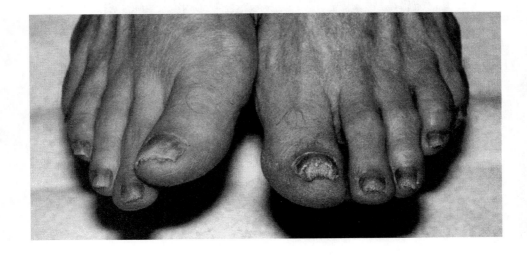

Picture 4- Onychocryptosis and paronychia

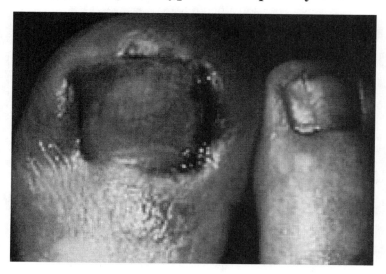

Picture 5- Koilonychia

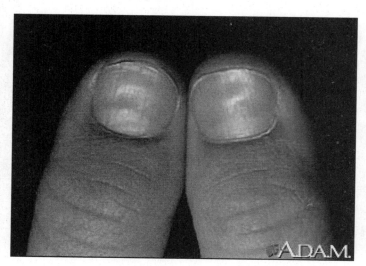

Picture 6- Beau Lines

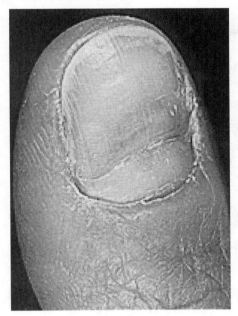

Picture 7- Clubbed Nails

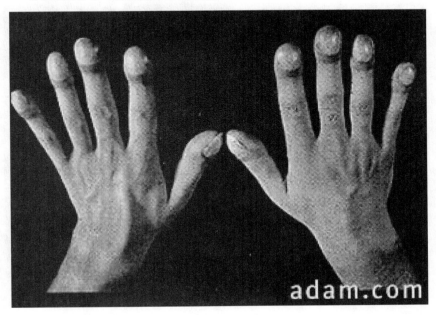

Picture 8- Psoriasis

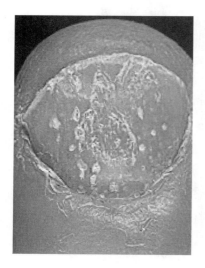

Picture 9- Periungual Warts

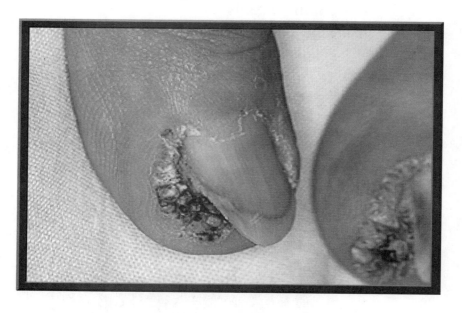

Picture 10- Lichen Planus

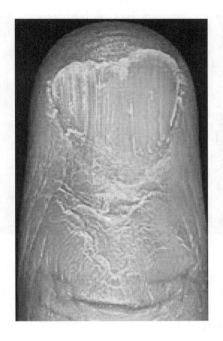

Picture 11- Bunion

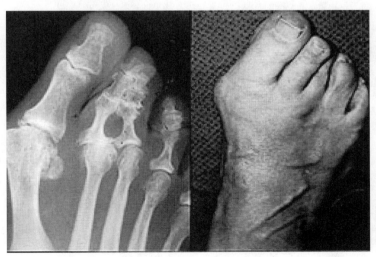

Picture 12- Hammertoe, mallot toe, and claw toe

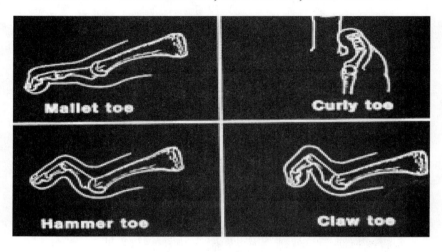

Picture 13- Heloma molle

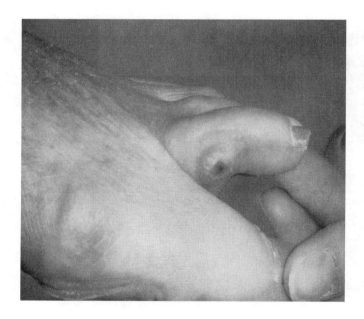

Picture 14- Plantar Fascia

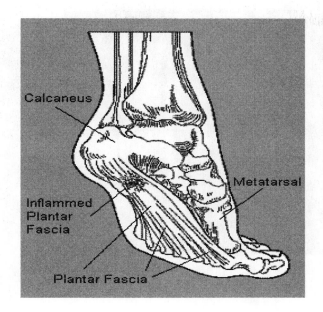

Picture 15- Achilles tendon stretch

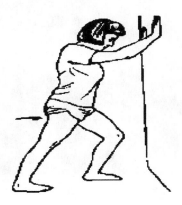

Picture 16- Psoriatic Arthritis

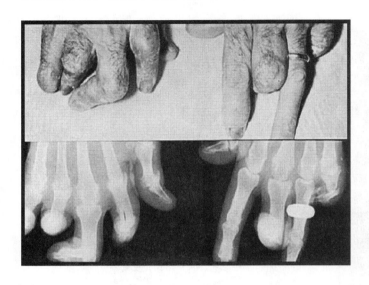

Picture 17- Charcot Joint

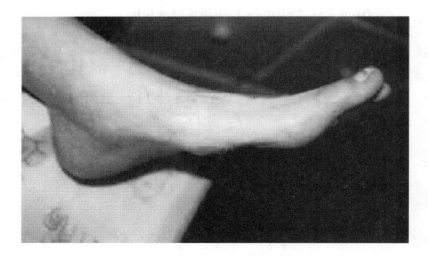

Picture 18- Charcot Joint with ulceration

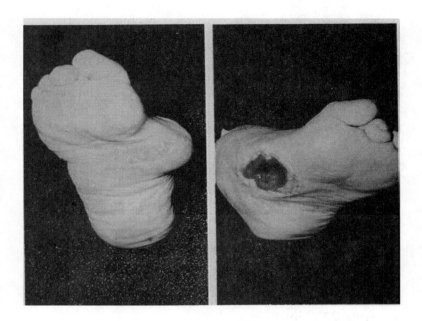

Picture 19- Plantar Wart

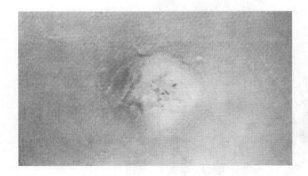

Picture 20- Ankle ligaments

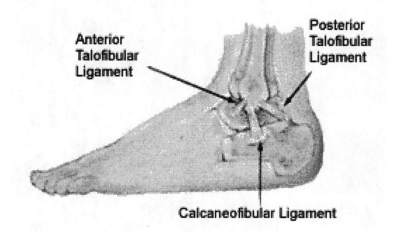

Anterior Talofibular Ligament

Posterior Talofibular Ligament

Calcaneofibular Ligament

Picture 21- Neuroma

Morton's Neuroma

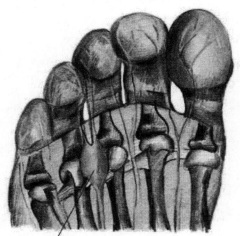

Neuroma

Picture 22- Chronic Venous Insufficiency

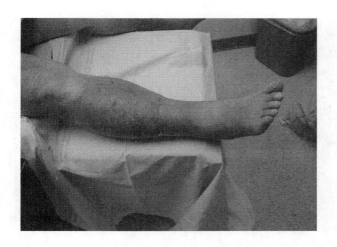

Picture 23- Arterial Disease

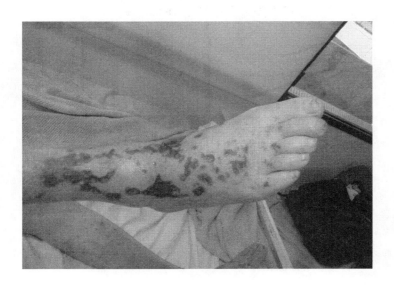

Picture 24- Lymphedema

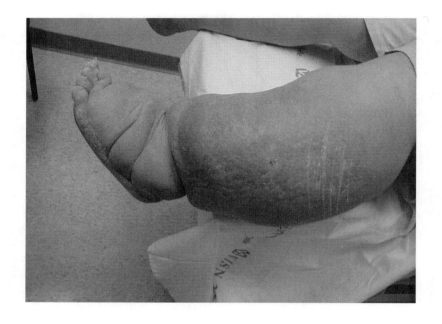

Picture 25- Diabetic ulceration

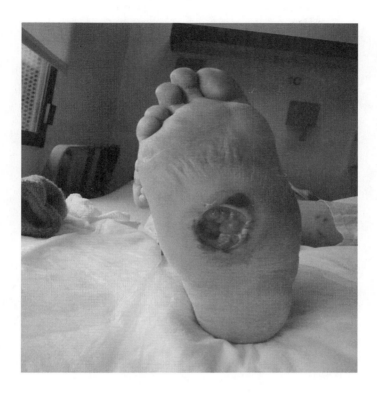

Bibliography

Plantar Fascitis. Arthroscopy.com
http://www.arthroscopy.com

www.healthlinkusa.com
psoriasis

Ribotsky, Bret "Charcot Jt"
www.Doctorbret.com

Agale, Melanie "Charcot joints."
Curtin Health Science Dept of Podiatry Encyclopedia
http://wwwcurtin.edu.au/curtin/dept/physio/podiatryencycl
opedia/charcot/

"Anatomy." Podiatry Forum. Podiatry Channel
http://www.podiatrychannel.com/anatomy/

"Morton's Neuroma"
http://www.podiatrychannel.com/mortonneuroma/

Goldberg, Charlie M.D., "A Practical Guide to Clinical
Medicine." The Lower Extremities
http://medicine.ucsd.edu/clinicalmed/upper.htm.

www.sportsmedicine.com

Walter, Stacy, Plantar Verrucae. Stevens and Lowe 1995
http://www.curtin.edu.au/curtin/dept./physio/podiatry/ency
clopedia/plantarverrucae/content.html

http://www.whymyfoothurts.com/conditions/rheumatoidart
hritis.html

Tanzi, Elizabeth M.D., Scher, Richard M.D.
Managing Common Nail Disorders in Active Patients and
Athletes. Physician and Sports Medicine Journal
Volume 27 No. 9 Sept. 1999

Onychomycosis
www.skinsite.com

Hammertoe, mallot toe, claw toe, onychocryptosis, bunion
Galluzzo Foot and Ankle Clinic
www.footdoc-il.com

Heloma molle
Dr. Michael Zapf, Dr. Darren Payne
www.zfootdoc.com

Koilonychia
Medline Plus health information
National Library of Medicine